Your
THYROID
SOLUTION

A Breakthrough System To
Eliminate Thyroid Problems
Without Medication or Surgery

DR. ROOSEVELT SMITH, D.C.
DR. CLIFTON MAYS, D.C.

First Edition

Printed in the U.S.A.

ISBN-13: 978-1544985909
ISBN-10: 1544985908

TABLE OF CONTENTS

Introduction

If you are like most people, you may not usually spend much time thinking about your thyroid. Among the long list of health concerns you may have for yourself or your loved ones, the thyroid is not one of the first health concerns that you may have. In fact, it's probably safe to say that the thyroid is largely overlooked in the standard discussions of public health, and that it is something of a mystery. But surprisingly, thyroid problems affect millions of people each day, and there are potentially serious side effects to consider when a thyroid problem is encountered.

In the media today, what are some of the health concerns that you hear about on a regular basis? Most likely, you have heard a lot about cancer, obesity, diabetes, a variety of viruses, and others. Of course, all of those are serious issues, and they mostly warrant the attention that they receive. However, thyroid problems are both serious and extremely common, meaning there is a good chance that either yourself or someone close to you will be affected by a thyroid problem at some point in time. Understanding exactly what it is that your thyroid does, and why it is important, is an important part of monitoring your health on an ongoing basis.

Some Background on the Thyroid

Unless you are a doctor or have spent time studying, you may not know much at all about the thyroid. The thyroid, which is a gland that is found in the front of your neck, is responsible for a variety of functions that influence many of the systems in your body. Thyroid hormones are produced within your thyroid gland, and those hormones are then sent through the blood throughout the body, where they do their part to keep your system working properly. Obviously, if there is a problem in the thyroid, there will be an impact on how your body is working, and you may notice the development of other health issues and de effects as a result (more on this later).

There is a close connection between the pituitary gland at the base of your brain and the functioning of your thyroid. The pituitary gland is responsible for telling the thyroid whether it needs to produce more or less hormones in order to keep your system in balance. One of the key nutrients that allows your thyroid to work as it should, is iodine. You need to have a sufficient level of iodine in your body. Iodine is used in the production of thyroid hormone, so having too little in your body can create a problem. In the modern world, iodine has been added to salt as a way of delivering it to people as part of their regular diet. For most people, iodine deficiency is not a problem as long as a 'regular' diet is being consumed.

The operation of your thyroid is closely tied to your metabolism, meaning a thyroid that is working improperly can have an adverse affect on how fast or slow your system works on a daily basis. This functioning of your body's metabolism can have a profound impact on how you feel each day, as you may notice a number of symptoms that leave you feeling something short of your best when you have a metabolism that isn't functioning at a normal rate.

Hyper and Hypo

As mentioned previously, the thyroid does not receive nearly as much attention as many other parts of the body, even though it has a major impact on your health. However, if you have heard anything at all about thyroid problems, you are probably familiar with the following two words – hypothyroidism, and hyperthyroidism. These are the two most common diseases that will come to mind with talking about the thyroid, and they combine to affect millions of people on a daily basis. If you have either hypothyroidism or hyperthyroidism, you are likely to experience a collection of health problems that can range from bothersome complaints to rather severe health issues.

As the name would suggest, people who are affected by hyperthyroidism have an overactive thyroid, which is producing more hormone than the body actually needs. While it might seem like a good problem to have too much of this important hormone, an overload of thyroid hormone can cause a number of issues within your system. Some of the potential problems experienced in those facing hyperthyroidism are as follows –

- Difficulty when trying to focus even on simple tasks
- Elevated heart rate
- Difficulty sleeping
- Unwanted weight loss
- Consistently feeling warm when others around you are not warm
- Ongoing feelings of nervousness

Of course, those are just some of the symptoms that could be experienced in a person with hyperthyroidism. The exact list of symptoms will vary from person to person, but most people will report at least some degree of discomfort or irritability when they have too much thyroid hormone in their blood.

On the other side of the equation, hypothyroidism is diagnosed as the underproduction of thyroid hormone. If your thyroid isn't meeting the demands of your body for the hormone, you will find that your entire system 'slows down' and you encounter problems that are largely the opposite of those seen above. Individuals with hypothyroidism are likely to see some of the symptoms below –

- Regularly feeling tired
- Slow heart rate

- Dry skin
- Feeling cold when those around you are not cold
- Unexpected weight gain despite healthy diet and consistent exercise
- Problems with constipation

As you can see, the problems experienced with this kind of thyroid problem are just as serious, although somewhat different, from the issues listed for those with hyperthyroidism. Rather than just ignoring these frustrating and uncomfortable symptoms of a thyroid problem, it is best to have your condition examined by a doctor in order to truly get to the bottom of the issue as quickly as possible.

Throughout the rest of this book, we are going to take a closer look at a variety of topics related to the thyroid. There are obviously some kinds of disconnect between public understanding of this important health issue and the actual prevalence of the problem, so it is important that you are educated on just how it is that thyroid problems go undetected in such a large number of people. Also, we will dive into the various ways that your thyroid can develop problems, and how those problems are likely to affect your day to day life. In the end, we hope you are left with a clear understanding of why the thyroid is so important, what can go wrong with its operation, and what steps you should take to address any thyroid problems that may be affecting your health. Thanks for reading, and let's get started.

CHAPTER ONE

Why Do I Feel Sick?

The simple question that is used for the title of this chapter is often the one that leads people down a path of discovering that they have some sort of thyroid problem. Unexplained health problems are always concerning, so many people head to the doctor to figure out exactly what is going on that has them feeling 'not quite right'. Unfortunately, the resulting diagnosis does not always point back to the thyroid, which can mean the patient is in for a long and frustrating process before they are able to finally get answers that can lead to improvement in their health.

Early on, we can see how the issue of under-education when it comes to the thyroid is a bit of a problem in terms if diagnosis and eventual treatment. With many other health issues, the patient will immediately be concerned about specific symptoms that point to a likely cause. For instance, there are symptoms that are often exhibited by individuals with diabetes, and these symptoms are well-known and recognized. Even before heading to the doctor, someone who hasn't been feeling well due to symptoms related to diabetes will already have a good idea of what is happening. In fact, they may tell the doctor straight away that they suspect a diabetic condition is the underlying cause.

This same pattern does not play out often when it comes to thyroid problems. Since thyroid issues are not usually on a patients' 'radar' when they head in for a doctor appointment, there is a good chance that this cause of health problems will be overlooked entirely. Thyroid issues are simply not as well-known or well-understood by the general public as are other health concerns, therefore this crucial gland is rarely considered when an individual begins to feel ill. Of course, given the incredible number of people who are dealing with some degree of thyroid problems at the moment, it is about time that this changed. People need to understand just how powerful the thyroid gland is in the daily operation of the body. Once there is greater understanding of the importance of the thyroid, there is a good chance that there will be an increased understanding to look to it as a solution to mysterious health problems.

A Wide Range of Signs

One of the reasons that the thyroid is often overlooked is due simply to the wide range of symptoms that can result from thyroid problems. The symptoms are greatly varied from patient to patient, meaning it is hard to locate a pattern that will immediately point to the thyroid as being the cause of poor health.

To help you better understand the many symptoms that could come to the surface when the thyroid is not functioning correctly, we have compiled a list below of some of the possible symptoms that you or someone you love may be experiencing. Of course, there are many other possible symptoms that could take place in a given individual, so this should not be considered an exhaustive list.

- **Feeling tired.** This is likely one of the most-common symptoms of a thyroid problem. When your thyroid isn't producing enough hormone (hypothyroidism), you are likely to still feel tired when you get up in the morning. Unfortunately, in the modern world, many people are accustomed to feeling tired simply due to being too busy and not getting enough sleep. Therefore, although this is a symptom that is commonly seen, it is usually one that is just attributed to lifestyle rather than a health condition.

- **Depression.** Feeling depressed is another common symptom that can come along with hypothyroidism. Of course, just as with feeling tired, this is not a condition that is considered rare in the modern world. Millions deal with depression on a daily basis, and most of those people can attribute those feelings to something other than a thyroid problem. However, it is believed that there is a connection between depression and low thyroid hormone levels, so don't overlook this potential warning sign.

- **Anxiety.** This symptom is very much on the other end of the spectrum from depression. If you are feeling anxious and 'jittery' throughout much of the day, you might have too much thyroid hormone running through your body. Just as having too little of this important hormone can lead to feeling down, having too much available can leave you too far 'up' – and you might not be able to relax as a result.

- **Loss of mental sharpness.** This point can be a difficult one to pin down, but it is certainly frustrating if you have to go through day to day life without your usual mental acuity. When you just can't quite think as clearly as you would usually, or when you are suddenly forgetful, you may be dealing with a thyroid problem. Both hypo and hyperthyroidism can lead to issues with brain function.

- **Lost sex drive.** A declined interest in sex may have something to do with a lack of thyroid hormone in your body as well. Often, it is the cumulative effect of other thyroid problem symptoms like lacking energy and feeling depressed that may leave you in no mood for sexual activity.

- **Weight gain.** Again, this is another problem that is hard to pin down to strictly a thyroid problem because there are so many other potential issues at work here. Are you gaining weight because of a thyroid issue, or because you have become less active in recent months? Or maybe you are eating more without noticing? Obviously, the issue of weight is a sensitive and complex one, which is why it is not always attributed to an underactive thyroid, which could in fact be the problem all along.

- **Infertility.** If you have been trying to get pregnant for some time with no luck, it is possible that the thyroid is at the heart of the matter. An improperly functioning thyroid – one that is producing either too much hormone or not enough – can interfere with the ovulation process, one that is obviously necessary for pregnancy. Those who feel like they have 'tried everything' when it comes to fertility problems should take the time to look at the possibility of a thyroid issue.

- **Dry skin.** This last point on our list is a health condition that you likely won't think much about when it pops up, but it can certainly be frustrating and uncomfortable to deal with if it persists. Dry skin is often itchy and does not help one to look their best, and the underlying cause of the condition can be hypothyroidism. However, most people associate this problem with other factors, such as the weather, age, diet or a host of other factors, which in turn means that it is often not seem as a symptom for thyroid trouble.

As you can see, the list of potential symptoms stemming from a thyroid problem is impressively long, and the above points are only a small sample of the many ways that this health issue can be manifested on a daily basis. In general, you can think about it this way – when your thyroid is under producing, your system as a whole will be working too slowly and the symptoms that result will represent that change (such as weight gain, depression). On the other hand, too much thyroid hormone can cause your system to work too fast, and the symptoms will swing the other way (anxiety, weight loss, etc.). Most important, however, is the fact that you need to keep the thyroid in mind if your health should take a negative turn. Most people don't consider thyroid problems when they have a health concern, but it is very possible that this important gland could be at the root of your issues. At the very least, the thyroid should be investigated any time there are unexplained health problems at hand.

The Obesity Epidemic

So, what do you do when you start to notice that you aren't quite feeling 'right' on a day to day basis? You make an appointment to see your doctor, of course. Most people will simply start with their general practice physician or family doctor, as that is the easiest place to get started with an exam. You make an appointment to see the doctor, you tell him or her about your symptoms, and the process goes from there. Unfortunately, while the medical industry today is able to do many great things and solve many challenging health problems, going into this process with a thyroid problem may not lead to the answers you need to find your way back to full health.

There are a couple of common problems that frequently lead doctors today to miss on the diagnosis of a thyroid problem. The first problem is the overwhelming number of overweight, lethargic people who are present in our society today. Simply put, doctors see patients complaining about weight and energy problems on a daily basis. These symptoms are not at all rare in society these days, and often the problem has nothing to do with the thyroid. Frequently, individuals are overweight and tired simply due to a combination of a poor diet and a lack of exercise. These people don't need treatment for their thyroid – they need a better health plan overall, and the symptoms they are experiencing will likely fade away. This increase in the population with weight issues has created a "blind spot" for many family doctors when it comes to thyroid disorders.

If you were a doctor, you can understand why it would be easy to lump all of these patients into the same general category.

The diagnosis seems so simple – get some exercise, eat a healthier diet, and watch your symptoms improve. Gladly, for many people, that will be exactly how it works. Unfortunately, it isn't going to play out that way for everyone. Some people – those who are facing a thyroid function problem rather than just a diet/exercise problem – are going to find that even with an improved diet and more activity, they still are unable to shake their symptoms.

The issue of obesity is the first hurdle in the way of more accurate and more timely thyroid diagnoses. Since obesity is an issue that is faced by millions of people, and it shares many symptoms with those who are suffering from an underactive thyroid, it is easy for health professionals to look at all of these patients in the same light. And, since the patient probably isn't thinking about a thyroid problem in the first place, they are likely to go along with the initial recommendation of the typical diet and exercise combination to fix the problem. This fact alone can start you down a road to ill health, that can be difficult to recover from.

Mental Health

In addition to obesity, mental health is another problem that has become more and more prevalent in recent years. Millions struggle with mental health on a daily basis, with the challenges they face running the spectrum from relatively minor to extremely serious. Here again, we see an overlap with problems of the thyroid, and another hurdle that must be cleared on the way toward a successful and accurate diagnosis.

As was mentioned in a previous section, some of the symptoms of thyroid problems can be related to mental health. Most notably, both depression and anxiety can stem from problems of the thyroid, depending on whether your body is producing too much or not enough of the hormone. Either way, an incorrect level of thyroid hormone in your body has the potential to lead you down a path of mental health issues, meaning you could find yourself going to the doctor to seek help at some point in the near future.

When you do go look for help, you are going to find the same problem that is seen in the case of obesity. Since healthcare professionals see so many patients who are suffering from a degree of depression or anxiety, it is not commonly considered to test the thyroid at this point. There are plenty of other issues that can lead to mental health challenges, such as stress at work, strained relationships, loss of a loved one, and more. Certainly not all people who have depression or anxiety are dealing with a thyroid issue, so the thyroid is not the first place to 'look' for a solution. However, it is going to be the correct solution for a percentage of patients, so it is important that it is at least considered as a possibility when depression and anxiety are present.

Getting There – Eventually

It's not that thyroid problems are never diagnosed in those who suffer from them – they are. However, it is the path that has to be taken to get there which can be frustrating, expensive, time consuming, and more. If you are feeling less than your best on a daily basis, you want to be able to get back to life 'as usual' as quickly as possible. When you get passed around from doctor to doctor for test after test, however, that isn't going to happen. If it takes many months or even years before you are diagnosed with the thyroid issue that has been causing problems all along, that really can't be seen as a victory. Only when thyroid problems are diagnosed both accurately and quickly can we feel good about having control over this common health concern.

CHAPTER TWO

Tests That Hurt Millions

When you go in to a medical facility to have tests completed, there is just one goal – to come to an accurate diagnosis of the underlying health problems. Of course, no one likes to go into the doctor's office or hospital for tests, but it is often necessary when you can't quite figure out what is wrong. In order to get to the bottom of your issues and have a treatment plan put in place that has a chance to be successful, you need to go through certain tests as recommended by your doctor.

As you would expect, that is also the case when it comes to the thyroid. If your doctor does suspect that there may be a thyroid problem at play in your case, he or she may choose to have your thyroid tested in order to determine how it is functioning. Usually, this means having one of two tests completed – either the TSH test, or the Free T4 test. While these tests take different approaches, they each have the same end result in mind – to find out how your thyroid is working, and what can be done to correct any problems that may exist.

TSH Test

Perhaps the single most-commonly used thyroid test is known as the TSH test. TSH stands for Thyroid-Stimulating Hormone, which is basically the hormone responsible for telling your thyroid what to do. This entire process starts in the brain itself. Part of the brain known as the hypothalamus releases a hormone known as TRH (thyroid releasing hormone), which is a trigger for the pituitary gland to release TSH, which then in turn tells the thyroid to take action. So, by testing for levels of TSH, doctors can determine how much work the thyroid is being asked to do, and then make an evaluation on whether it is working too hard, functioning correctly, or not working hard enough.

The test itself it simple enough – it can be completed through a basic blood draw. You will be asked to give a blood sample, which will then be tested, and the results will provide a TSH reading that is compared to a chart or range with established values for healthy thyroid production. Your doctor will give you the results of the test, along with their evaluation of how the results look with regard to the operation of your thyroid. While the established ranges for the results of a TSH test will help you determine how well the thyroid is working, your doctor will also be able to use judgment based on other factors in your specific case to decide if treatment is necessary.

Free T4 Test

The other option for thyroid testing is known as the Free T4 test. T4 is one of the two specific hormones produced by your thyroid – it is also known as thyroxine. You need to have an appropriate amount of T4, along with the other hormone, T3, in order to keep your system running properly. Along with testing the level of TSH in your blood to evaluate the function of your thyroid, a doctor may decide to test for Free T4 (often times, your doctor may test for both).

This test is called 'Free T4' because it is looking for the thyroxine in your blood that is 'free', rather than the thyroxine that is already attached to protein. If you test only for total T4, which includes that attached to protein, the results of the test can be misleading because of the varying amounts of protein which may be present in your system. Therefore, testing only the free and active T4 is considered a more accurate way to measure the level of this hormone in the blood. Again, the results of this test will be compared to an expected range to determine whether or not your body is producing an appropriate level of T4.

The Problems

So, what it is that is so wrong with these tests? Of course, they work just fine, and can be used to gain an understanding of how the thyroid is functioning in the body. However, they are only a snapshot of just one moment in time, and they only represent a portion of the overall picture of hormone production that needs to be considered. It is often possible for you to have a problem with your thyroid and yet still 'pass' these tests. When the numbers come back within the given range – even if they are only barely within that range – your doctor may decide to move on to look for other problems while prematurely setting aside the idea of a thyroid issue.

Unfortunately, thyroid testing is not taken as seriously as testing for many other health problems, which leads to a massive problem of under-diagnosis. There are millions dealing with thyroid problems who either don't know that they have the problem, or that have been told they don't need to worry about correcting a hormone level that may be only slightly outside the truly functional levels. As long as your test falls somewhere within the spectrum that has been deemed acceptable, you are usually either told that nothing is wrong, or told to look for answers in other places around your body. At the end of the day, the only thing you want out of the process is to feel better and to get back to your normal life. If that doesn't happen because your thyroid test fails to get to the heart of the issue, you will have been let down by the system. And a sad fact is that millions of people are "stuck" here with little or no where else to turn to. This is one of the primary reasons that this book was created, so that you can have hope.

CHAPTER THREE

What are Normals?

The concept of normal values within the medical field is always something of a guessing game. That's not to say that the healthcare professionals who are working on solving these problems don't know what they are doing – they do – but it is simply difficult, if not impossible, to assign a range of normal values to something like a blood test when all people are so different and unique. Attempting to account for all of the different variables that can be in place during a test while establishing an acceptable range is a task that is required by the system, but not necessarily as useful as it should be.

At this point, the generally accepted range for a TSH test to indicate a healthy and properly functioning thyroid is between 0.5 and 5.0. If a TSH test, which is often the only test ordered by a doctor who wishes to check on thyroid operation, comes back within that range, the patient is generally considered to have a healthy thyroid. However, that range will vary from lab to lab and doctor to doctor, so one healthcare professional may deem a 4.8 test as healthy while another would not, for example. Quite obviously, it is concerning that there is not complete agreement across the medical field as to what range of TSH level should be considered healthy.

Over time, the range that is accepted has gotten wider and wider, meaning fewer and fewer people are diagnosed with a thyroid condition. Casting a wider 'healthy' net means that more and more people are going un-diagnosed, even when they are right on the edge of perhaps needing intervention to get their thyroid working properly once again (or for the first time). Rather than ordering more tests if someone is one the edge of one end of the range or the other, it is common to have a doctor simply move on from this concern to test for another potential problem that could be at the root of health issues. Not surprisingly, many people go around and around with more and more tests before winding up back at the idea that it may have been the thyroid that was the problem all along.

Optimal Rather Than Acceptable

It is the concept of simply trying to fit patients within a range that doesn't sit right with many people, including some within the healthcare industry. Rather than just taking a test result and plugging it into a range to see if it fits, wouldn't the better approach be to see how close to optimal each patient can become? Even if a patient falls within the acceptable range for a TSH test, for example, it seems to stand to reason that their health could be improved if they were able to move the test result numbers closer to an optimal level.

For instance, someone who receives a test result of 4.9 in the TSH test might be told by the doctor that they are in the healthy range – but they are only barely within that acceptable border. At that point, it is still very possible to have negative health outcomes as a result of a questionable thyroid. If that same person could be moved down into the 2 or 3 range, it seems an almost certainty that their overall health would be improved. This should be the goal at the end of the day – not just 'good enough', but as good as is possible. This is the concept behind optimal lab ranges.

When it comes to your health, you absolutely do not want to settle for just 'okay'. The difference between managing your symptoms just to get by each day and actually taking care of problems so that you can live happily for years to come is huge. You don't want to just be getting through each day, you want to be enjoying those days and thriving in them with whatever opportunities you have in front of you. Unfortunately, when it comes to something as important to your health as the thyroid, many medical practices do not take that same approach. The thyroid has been viewed through the lens of trying to make it 'good enough' for a long time, and that approach obviously isn't working. Millions fight thyroid problems and the associated side effects, meaning the way we have been approaching this health problem is failing.

Only when we settle for nothing less than optimal when it comes to thyroid health are we really going to be able to provide individuals with the outcome they desire. No one wants to feel just 'good enough' each day, but that is what will be the case if the thyroid is not taken more seriously as a driver of overall health. The concept of 'normal' is one that is driven by entities such as testing labs and insurance companies, but it doesn't necessarily match up with what is best for the health of each individual patient. Only if we are willing to go beyond 'normal' and drill down to what is optimal for an individual will we have the chance to gain a hold on the growing thyroid problem.

CHAPTER FOUR

Why Medicine Does Not Work

If you do have a thyroid test result that comes back outside of the expected or acceptable range, there is a good chance that you will be prescribed a medication to correct the problem. For those with hypothyroidism, the medicine that is most-commonly prescribed is called levothyroxine (the brand Synthroid is often ordered). You will likely be asked to take a set amount of this drug on a daily basis, with the goal of moving your thyroid back into a healthy range.

As long as you take your medicine as prescribed on a regular basis, there is a good chance that you will indeed be able to move your levels back into a healthier range. There will likely be a follow-up blood test done to see if the drug has had its intended effect. As long as you are now within a healthy range on the TSH test, that will likely be the end of any thyroid treatment you will be recommended to receive. Your doctor will tell you to continue on taking the same dose of the medication, and you may be asked to check in for a new test from time to time to make sure the drug is continuing to have the desired effect on the lab values.

On the surface, this sounds great – your thyroid is back into an acceptable range, you only have to take a small pill each day, and you don't even have to spend all that much money on the medicine. A great outcome for all involved? Not necessarily. Sure, your lab tests may look great now that you have begun taking medication, but there may be one small problem remaining – you still may feel sick.

How could that be? How could you still feel sick when you now have your thyroid levels back within a healthy, normal range? There are a number of potential problems at work here. First, it is important to remember that the TSH test is not actually testing the function of your thyroid – it is testing for the hormone that is being sent to your thyroid to tell it to work. There are still many other complex functions involved in the overall workings of the thyroid hormone system, including the conversion of T4 into T3. If there is something else along the line that is wrong with your thyroid system as a whole, you still may be having those same old side effects like weight gain, depression, lack of energy, and more.

Naturally, this can be quite frustrating. Your doctor will likely tell you that nothing is wrong with your thyroid now that your tests are within what is considered a normal range, but you won't really believe it based on the way that you feel. If the thyroid is now working properly, why don't you feel better? It is easy to become tired of 'playing the game' when it comes to thyroid testing and medication, when you continue to be told that everything is fine despite the symptoms you are experiencing.

Not a Correction

By its very nature, medicine is not working to correct the underlying problem that you are experiencing with your health. Rather, it is only helping you to manage the symptoms that are experienced on a day to day basis. In this case, taking a drug like levothyroxine is simply going to artificially supplement the lacking thyroid hormone that is not being produced by your body. Surely for some, this may be a better situation than taking no action at all, but it really doesn't get to the heart of the problem. You don't really want to keep taking these pills for the rest of your life to manage symptoms and get by – you want to solve the problem and move on once and for all.

Whenever possible, the ideal outcome in a healthcare situation is to reach a solution that does not need to be treated on an ongoing basis. Rather than taking thyroid medication for the rest of your life, you would love to be able to reach a point where your thyroid is working properly on its own with no chemical intervention. Unfortunately, that is really not the way modern medicine works in most cases. Instead, we are told to simply keep taking our medicine to treat the symptoms and side effects, without keeping an eye toward an actual solution. There will be more about this issue discussed later in the book.

CHAPTER FIVE

Hypothyroidism

Hypothyroidism is extremely common (more common than hyperthyroidism), and it occurs most commonly in women (although it certainly can be found in men as well). If you suspect that you have a thyroid problem, and you have tests done to investigate the function of your thyroid, you could wind up being diagnosed with this condition. Of course, you will not be alone – this is a diagnosis that has been received by millions of people over the years, as hypothyroidism is a condition that affects many people in a variety of ways.

One of the disappointing and frustrating things that you are likely to experience upon your diagnosis is the lack of specific information that will be provided when you are told that you have hypothyroidism. In fact, that will likely be the end of the diagnosis. You will be told that your tests indicate an underactive thyroid, and you will probably be prescribed some medication, which is meant to treat the problem. After a period of time, you will return for another test to see if the medicine is having the intended effect. If so, that will likely be the end of the process (and you will be told to continue taking the medicine).

With all of that said, diagnosing someone with hypothyroidism is quite the general statement that really need more specifics in order to have any meaning or significance. Think about it this way – if a doctor informed you that you 'have cancer', what would your first question be? Of course, you would ask, 'what kind of cancer do I have'? That same question should be asked in reference to hypothyroidism, but sadly, it is rarely even considered. Most people, understandably, follow along with the suggestion from the doctor to take the standard medication, and they hope that it will take care of their challenging symptoms.

In reality, there are six different types of hypothyroidism. Rather than all being treated as the same thing, which is largely what happens in today's healthcare world, they should be treated uniquely based on the symptoms, blood tests and side effects of each. The way that hypothyroidism reveals itself in people varies wildly, yet the standard medical treatment that is offered doesn't vary at all. This antiquated plan for treating hypothyroidism clearly isn't working well, based on the number of people who still struggle with this condition on a daily basis. If you have been diagnosed with hypothyroidism and you are not sure that the treatment prescribed is actually having a positive impact on your health, you may want to take a closer look at how your condition is coming about. Depending on the type of hypothyroidism that you have, and the symptoms that you are experiencing, you may need to change your course of action in order to reach a desirable outcome.

Over the past several decades – 50 years or more – there has been a tremendous amount of change and development in the world of medicine. Illnesses that were once difficult or impossible to cure have been conquered, and the overall health of the public has greatly improved. With that said, there hasn't been much change at all in the way we treat hypothyroidism. The treatment for this condition hasn't really changed at all in that time, and the result is health outcomes that are largely disappointing to those who are affected. Although standard medical treatment remains unchanged, there is a movement in today's healthcare to develop better medicine, with the goal of understanding the true cause of thyroid issues. This movement is leading to a path of improved health outcomes as well as providing patients with more accurate, more specific diagnoses. This book is your introduction to today's modern healthcare movement.

In the following chapters, we are going to go through each of the six different types of hypothyroidism. Hopefully, by reviewing these chapters one by one, you can gain a better understanding for the various ways that hypothyroidism can become a problem in your life, and how it works 'behind the scenes'. Being informed is the best way to make smart decisions about your health moving forward, and we know that the content below is a step in that direction.

CHAPTER SIX

Primary Hypothyroidism

In many ways, this can be thought of as 'standard' hypothyroidism. In this case, it really is the failing of your thyroid that is leading to the problems that you are experiencing. Rather than a cause and effect 'chain' like some of the types of hypothyroidism can offer, this form is basic and straightforward in nature. Quite simply, your thyroid is not producing enough hormone, and it needs to pick up the pace in order to get your health back on track.

You can think about this kind of hypothyroidism as your thyroid simply getting lazy on the job. Rather than doing what it is supposed to do – which is to produce T4 and T3 hormone at a high enough rate to run all of your body's functions, it is falling down on the job and falling short of needed production. In the end, you don't have enough thyroid hormone running through your blood on a regular basis, and your health begins to deteriorate. You may find that you gain weight without changing your habits, you may have low energy levels, you might feel depressed, and more. There are countless ways in which low thyroid hormone problems can manifest themselves in your day to day life (many of which were covered earlier).

When your body realizes that there is an insufficient amount of the thyroid hormone in your blood, it will respond in an effort to rectify the problem. That action takes the form of the pituitary gland working over time, sending extra TSH to the thyroid in order to encourage it to get started once again. That extra TSH that is being produced in the pituitary gland is what will likely be measured in your blood test, and it is what will tell your doctor that your thyroid is not doing enough to keep you healthy. When this kind of primary hypothyroidism is in place, your TSH levels will read well above the optimal amount when your blood is tested, and action will need to be taken in order to bring them back down and improve the overall balance of thyroid in your blood.

In this case, and this case alone (with the possible exception of Hashimoto's, which we will cover later), patients may respond well to hormone replacement therapy, or HRT. For most people with primary hypothyroidism, the HRT that they receive is the Synthroid medication we discussed earlier. This is the kind of treatment that was mentioned above, and it is the treatment that is far and away the most common and most popular for thyroid issues. Since the problem is direct and simple in nature – the thyroid isn't producing enough hormone to fil the body's needs, you can use the prescribed hormone replacement to fill in the gap. Using HRT isn't as much of a stop-gap in this case because it pretty much addresses the problem directly at the core level. Your body doesn't have enough thyroid hormone because the thyroid is refusing to produce an adequate amount, so that amount is filled in with medicine.

In these cases, this kind of treatment is effective and the patient will see a great reduction – if not elimination – in his or her symptoms. Since the medicine is relatively affordable and easy to take, most people do not mind staying on it as long as future blood tests show that the thyroid hormone in the blood is back near an optimal level. Ongoing checkups will be necessary to make sure the thyroid levels in the blood remain in an appropriate range, but for the most part the patient should be able to go on living without too much concern about their thyroid issue. Although this can be an effective treatment regime for primary hypothyroidism, only small amounts of people truly have "primary hypothyroidism" as their only diagnosis. This is why millions of people taking medication still have issues and are then told to just live with it. It is also important to understand that a person can have more than one "type" of hypothyroidism as the problem. This leads us to addressing the next "type of hypothyroidism".

CHAPTER SEVEN

Hypothyroidism Secondary to Pituitary Hypofunction

This next type of hypothyroidism is one where the thyroid isn't actually the main culprit - meaning an alternative treatment will be necessary in order to get things back on track. Treating this problem with hormone therapy or Synthroid in this case would be missing the point. Rather than dealing directly with the thyroid when it isn't the problem to begin with, many would argue that it makes more sense to address the root cause of the issue that is leading to an insufficient supply of thyroid hormone.

In this case, we are talking about a pituitary gland problem which is creating an issue with thyroid levels. Specifically, we are looking at an underperforming pituitary which is leaving you without enough TSH to trigger an appropriate response from your thyroid. If the thyroid isn't being told that it needs to produce more hormone, it naturally isn't going to do so – meaning you will be short on T4 and T3, but it really won't be the fault of your thyroid itself. Following the chain of events back to the start, it is the pituitary gland that is causing the problems, and the low thyroid levels that are making you feel sick are simply the manifestation of those original issues.

To correct the actual root cause of the problem in this case, you will need to address the matter of why the pituitary gland is failing to send enough TSH toward your thyroid in the first place. That is the real problem here, and that is the problem that should be solved as quickly and effectively as possible. If you are able to get your pituitary gland back to producing an appropriate level of the hormones that it is responsible for, it would not be necessary to treat your symptoms with HRT or other supplement for your thyroid.

There are a number of symptoms which can be attributed to pituitary hypofunction, including the following -

- Stomach pain and loss of appetite
- Extreme thirst
- Headache (especially in the mornings)
- Sensitivity to cold
- Stiffness in your joints

Obviously, those are only a few of the many possible symptoms that you could experience when your pituitary gland is struggling to keep up with hormone demand. To confirm that you actually have a problem with your pituitary gland rather than just your thyroid, you will need to undergo a blood test. Among the various potential causes for this condition include a tumor, prior brain surgery, brain bleeding, conditions present at birth, interference in the pituitary-adrenal axis and more. In some cases, the precise cause of the condition may never be known.

One of the most-common causes of pituitary malfunction, and one that was not included in the previous paragraph, is stress and fatigue. When you are regularly stressed as a result of your day to day life – whether due to stress from your job, personal life, or something else entirely – you will run the risk of fatiguing your pituitary gland to the point where it is no long holding up its end of the bargain. Stress manifests itself in a number of negative ways throughout the body, and this is yet another one to add to the list.

Potentially, you could improve the function of your pituitary gland simply by reducing the amount of stress that you feel on a day to day basis.

Another issue to keep in mind when it comes to the function of the pituitary gland is the matter of insulin levels. Usually associated with diabetes, fluctuating insulin levels can have a profound impact on the operation of the rest of your body as well, including your glands. When your glucose levels are frequently moving up and down throughout the day, your glands can become fatigued and slow down to a point where they are no longer producing the hormones necessary to keep up with your regular bodily functions. By taking steps to even out those fluctuations –

which will be good for your health in other ways, as well – you can take a big step towards giving your pituitary gland a chance to do what it is supposed to be doing.

CHAPTER EIGHT

Thyroid Under-Conversion

One of the components of the thyroid hormone process that is frequently overlooked is the conversion of T4 hormone into T3 hormone. T4 is considered the "inactive" form of thyroid hormone and in order for the hormone to be effective in the body, it has to be converted to the "active" form or T3. This is a vital step in the process, but it is a step that doesn't always function as it should. When your body is not properly converting T4 into T3, you may find that your system is not running as it should even though the thyroid gland is making plenty of T4 to start with. This is again a case for understanding and testing the entire process of how the thyroid gland works to understand what is going on, and why. If you were to treat this problem by simply taking a synthetic thyroid medication, all you would be doing is producing excess T4 – you wouldn't be doing anything toward solving the real problem of turning T4 into T3.

Again in this case, stress can be at the heart of the issue. When you are dealing with ongoing stress that is taking a toll on your mind and body, it can be manifested in a number of ways. One such way is through chronic adrenal stress. Basically, your system is stressed from top to bottom, and it fails to perform as it should as a result. In terms of trying to convert T4 to T3, the problem is an excess amount of cortisol in your system. Too much cortisol will suppress the conversion of T4 to T3, making it seem like there may be a thyroid problem when the issue isn't actually with the thyroid itself at all.

Unfortunately, this is another way in which a thyroid problem can be misdiagnosed, or just missed altogether. With a standard thyroid blood test – the TSH variety – only levels of T4 are going to be observed. Since the levels of T4 have an effect on TSH production, but T3 does not, you could be led to believe that everything is fine with your thyroid hormone levels when you only undergo the standard thyroid tests. The TSH test very well may come back within the normal range due to the fact that you have plenty of T4 in your blood. What will have been missed, however, is the fact that you do not have enough T3, which is why you still don't feel well even though the blood test says that your thyroid levels are "normal" and you have nothing to worry about.

Solving thyroid under-conversion may be as simple as working to improve your chronic adrenal stress, which may be causing excess cortisol to get in the way of the conversion. Producing T4 in your thyroid is great, but only if that T4 is being converted to the T3 that you need to function properly on an ongoing basis. Without enough T3, you are going to have many of the symptoms that are commonly seen in those with hypothyroidism. However, this form of hypothyroidism is unique from the others we have looked at so far, and the others that are still to come. You shouldn't treat all forms of this condition in the same manner, because they stem from different places and each has its own unique solution.

CHAPTER NINE

Thyroid Over-Conversion and Decreased TBG

In just the same way that under-conversion from T4 to T3 can lead to problems, so too can problems arise when too much T4 is converted over into T3. This over-conversion problem leads to an overwhelming of the cells, again causing the body to operate at a level that is less than optimal. As you suspect, in order for everything in your system to be working correctly as far as the thyroid hormone is concerned, you need to have just the right amount of T4 turning into T3 – not too much, and not too little.

There is another element that plays a role in this equation, which is known as TBG, or thyroxine-binding globulin. As the name would indicate, this is a protein that binds with the thyroid hormone to carry it through the blood. When there isn't enough TBG in your system, the T4 that has converted to T3 will not have anywhere to attach, and there will be more of it running free in the bloodstream than is ideal. While this issue in and of itself is not necessarily a problem, it can lead to other issues, especially when it comes to trying to pin down exactly how well the thyroid itself is functioning.

So what is the cause of this problem? Again, it doesn't actually originate in the thyroid at all, but rather it can be related to insulin resistance. While this can be a problem in anyone, it is especially common to find in women. Insulin resistance is a problem frequently associated with diabetes, and yet it is also seen to cause problems here when it comes to the levels of thyroid hormone in the body.

Basically, insulin resistance means that your cells are not 'hearing' what the insulin in your body is trying to tell them. Ideally, the presence of insulin will alert your cells that more insulin is not needed, so no more (or at least, less) will be produced. In a person without diabetes, this is how the system works. However, when a diabetic condition or other issue is present, insulin resistance may cause trouble within the workings of this process. Instead of the insulin alerting the cells to its presence, those cells will not receive the message and more insulin than is needed will be created. That extra insulin is not needed, and it can cause problems in a number of ways.

One of the biggest problems extra insulin production can cause as it related to the thyroid is an increased testosterone level. When a women's testosterone level is increased higher than normal, there may as a result be a reduced level of TBG in the blood and too much free T3 running around as a result. So, again in this case, we see that a problem, which seems to be tied to the thyroid directly actually has a number of other underlying causes. In this case, it is insulin resistance that is often to blame for low TBG levels and high levels of T3 remaining free in the system. A treatment that targets the thyroid in this case wouldn't make a lot of sense, and the thyroid isn't doing anything wrong (at least, not as far as this condition is concerned). Rather, it is the matter of insulin resistance that is leading to trouble that comes back to the thyroid hormone. If you suffered from this condition, and you were able to straighten out the way your body responds to insulin, it very well may be that the thyroid problem would then take care of itself. This is also one of the "double-edged" swords in regard to obesity. Many doctors will address peoples "diabetes" issues and hope that it takes care of the person's weight issues, but if the thyroid is involved in their issue and no steps are taken to correct this "conversion" issue as well, the symptoms return and the weight issues continue. This is one of the dangerous cycles of disease that we see "mis-diagnosed" on a daily basis. So if weight issues have been a primary concern and you've taken steps to manage your insulin levels, it is time to check out your thyroid.

CHAPTER TEN

Thyroid Binding Globulin Elevation

That very same TBG that we discussed in the previous section can also produce a problem when there is too much of it available as opposed to too little. In fact, pretty much everything in this whole system of thyroid hormone production is a case of needing to be in perfect balance – when too much or too little of anything is present, problems can arise. Those problems might not seem major on their own, but they can begin to lead to varieties of side effects and symptoms which range from unpleasant to quite severe.

When there is too much TBG in the blood, there will in turn be a lack of free T3 because nearly all of it will have attached to TBG since that protein will be in such ample supply. With too much TBG flowing throughout your body, none of the T3 that is converted from T4 will even have a chance to get to the cells where it is needed and there is not enough hormone in the body that will remain free. In order to once again free up an appropriate level of T3 that can move throughout your body without being attached to a protein, you will need to successfully lower the level of TBG that you have available.

What is it that could cause TBG to be elevated in the first place? There are a couple of possibilities, specifically for women. The first is oral contraceptives. If you are taking an oral contraceptive, it is possible that a side effect of that medicine could be an elevated level of TBG. One result of taking oral contraceptives can be an elevated estrogen level, and high estrogen is often associated with your body creating more TBG than is necessary. Since many of the women in today's society have been on birth control for 30 or more years, this imbalance in estrogen can play a large role in how TBG levels are maintained.

Another possibility when dealing with high TBG is simply having estrogen replacement therapy. If your doctor has recommended estrogen replacement therapy for any reason, it is possible that those treatments are causing trouble within your TBG levels. Of course, before you simply stop with that therapy in order to help your TBG, you will need to consult with your doctor to figure out a solution that is going to best meet with all of your needs. There are occasionally treatments that conflict with each other in the healthcare world, and it is up to a qualified doctor to figure out how to bring them together in a way that will lead to a positive health outcome in the long run.

CHAPTER ELEVEN

Autoimmune Disorders

The autoimmune disorder that is typically associated with hypothyroidism is known as Hashimoto's Disease. Simply put, this is an autoimmune disorder where your immune system determines that it needs to attack your thyroid. Since your thyroid is under attack from your own system, it will be inflamed on a chronic basis, and likely will under produce thyroid hormone as a result. The most common group to suffer from this disease is middle-aged women, although is can appear in anyone. It is believed that Hashimoto's is actually the leading cause of hypothyroidism today. If fact, as many as 90% of cases of hypothyroidism are linked to an autoimmune disorder.

This is a disease that comes on slowly over time, so you may not notice the symptoms right away. Often, the only visible symptom – if there is a visible symptom at all – is a swelling in the front of your throat where the thyroid is located. As you would expect, the majority of the symptoms of an autoimmune disorder affecting your thyroid production are the same as they would be for any other form of hypothyroidism. Those include fatigue, weight gain, dry skin, sore muscles, depression, and more. Of course, you will not likely experience all of these symptoms, but you may encounter more than a few of them along the way.

Autoimmune diseases in general, including Hashimoto's any many others, are basically your body making a mistake. Rather than attacking the unwelcome cells that you need to get rid of in order to stay health, your body is mistakenly begins to use its immune system to attack healthy, needed cells such as the thyroid. It can be hard to diagnose an autoimmune disorder because of the many different side effects and various issues that can come up as a result of this type of problem. Also, since there are around 80 different autoimmune disorders which can affect the body, doctor's have their hands full when trying to pin down exactly what is causing a health problem.

One of the frustrating factors in dealing with an autoimmune disorder is that the cause is not known. While there are various theories that abound regarding what sort of things may be risk factors, the reality is that science does not yet know why your body chooses to attack specific healthy parts of itself rather than only fighting against unwanted and unneeded cells. In the case of Hashimoto's, being female greatly increases your odds of getting this disease, as does having another autoimmune disease and having Hashimoto's history within your family.

If you believe you are dealing with Hashimoto's disease it is important to understand that you may have other organs within your body, which are being attacked as well. As many as 50% - 60% of people who have Hashimoto's also have other organs in the body that are coming under attack regularly. These attacks fall into a number of categories, and can be associated with a number of other diseases, including the following –

- Pancreas – Diabetes
- Brain – Parkinson's, Alzheimer's, Dementia
- Intestine – Crohn's, IBS
- Joints – RA
- Uterus – Endometriosis
- Spine – Osteoporosis

As you can see, some of these diseases can be very serious in nature. Addressing any autoimmune problems that you may be having in your body is an important step to take as quickly as possible to ensure that you receive the best care possible in a timely fashion. The good news in regard to this condition is that there are specific blood tests that can determine if Hashimoto's disorder may be contributing to your thyroid issue. Although we stated earlier that autoimmune disorders are difficult to pin down, a doctor knowledgeable in thyroid dysfunction is much better able to narrow down the possible underlying causes.

CHAPTER 12

What Do I Do Now?

If you have read through this entire book, you should now have a great understanding of the important points related to hypothyroidism and the various effects that it can have on your life. While it is also possible to have your life impacted by hyperthyroidism, the majority of people who struggle with incorrect levels of thyroid hormone are going to be on the hypo end of the spectrum. As you now know, just saying that someone has hypothyroidism is a bit too general for any true understanding, as there are six different kinds of this health problem, and each has its own unique solution.

The first thing you should do about your potential thyroid problem is to take action. Nothing is going to get better if you just sit back and deal with your symptoms and side effects day after day. You should be able to get out of bed each morning feeling good about yourself and the day to come. If you are fighting with things like unexplained weight gain and lethargy, you need to take action to do something about those problems as quickly as possible. It is easy to dismiss your symptoms as being caused by another issue, perhaps even something that is your own fault. Many overweight individuals decide that they alone are to blame for their health problems, when that might not be the case at all.

It is important to be honest with yourself in this process, because that honesty is what will likely lead you to a solution in the end. Do you think that your symptoms are due to personal health choices that need to be improved, or is there something else at play? Obviously, someone who eats everything they want and never exercises is likely to gain weight. However, if you haven't really changed your habits and you continue to gain weight – or are unable to lose weight despite putting in a focused, consistent effort, you might be suffering from a thyroid problem.

The story is the same when it comes to things like feeling tired and not having enough motivation to get through your day. Are you getting enough sleep? If not, make sure to get plenty of sleep and monitor how your energy level changes. If you know you are getting plenty of quality sleep each night, you can cross that off the list and start to look for other causes of the lethargic feelings that you just can't shake.

One of the most important lessons that you can take from this book is simply to be aware of yourself, and aware of any changes that are taking place in your body. The way your body looks and feels is a reflection on your lifestyle, unless something else is interfering with the normal processes that should keep you running smoothly. So, a change in your body and the way it functions that cannot be explained by changes in your habits or lifestyle is likely going to be best explained by some form of disease or other health issue. If you are paying attention to your body, and listening to what it is telling you, it will be possible to take action quickly in order to get the answers you need.

The Right Doctor

Working your way toward health requires a partnership between yourself and the right doctor. While all doctors are put through rigorous schooling and training on their way to becoming physicians, not all practicing doctors have an equal amount of experience working with the thyroid. You want to be working with a doctor who is particularly experienced in this area in order to give yourself the best possible chance at finding a successful solution.

One of the important factors that you will benefit from when working with an experienced doctor who is familiar with thyroid problems is the willingness to try a variety of treatments and tests. As mentioned throughout this book, it is common for doctors to simply turn to the TSH test and then leave things alone from there. The entire diagnosis and medication plan is usually based on the number that is returned from the TSH test, but as you have read, thyroid problems are rarely that simple. In reality, it may take a number of tests and different medications or other treatments in order to get to the right place that allows you to feel your best. You want to be working with a doctor who is open-minded, experienced with the thyroid, and willing to listen to your input along the way. You know your body better than anyone else ever can, so be sure to make your feelings and thoughts known throughout the process. Your doctor should welcome your feedback, and if not, you should simply find one who will.

Once you do find a doctor with the thyroid experience that you are looking for and the willingness to try a number of approaches in order to reach a successful outcome, you should do your best to stick with that doctor for as long as possible. Building a long-term relationship with your physician is desirable because that doctor will be able to get to know you both as a patient and as a person. Familiarity frequently leads to better health outcomes in the long run, so make it a point to stick with your doctor – particularly as it relates to issues with your thyroid.

The Right Tests

Most people try to be 'good' patients when they go into the doctor's office. What does it mean to be a 'good' patient? Generally speaking, these are people who will follow directions, do as their told, and follow along with the doctor's advice. And, most of the time, that is a great way to approach healthcare. After all, the professionals that are treating you are educated and experienced, and they know far more about medicine and the human body than you do. However, that authority only goes so far, and at some point you need to be willing to step up and speak your mind for the best interest of your health.

One of those cases is when the time comes to test your thyroid. Now that you understand more about the system that produces thyroid hormone in your body, you should realize that a simple TSH test is not always going to be enough to get a true picture of the condition of your thyroid. Just testing TSH alone only takes a look at one specific part of the overall system that is working to keep your healthy. It is quite possible to have the results of this test look normal while the thyroid is actually not quite doing its job, as it should. In other words, just because your test results when blood work is done fall within the 'normal' range does not mean you are necessarily in a good place with your thyroid health.

If your doctor plans to only run a TSH test to evaluate the condition of your thyroid, consider asking about the possibility of running other tests as well. As long as you are taking the time and effort to go to doctor's appointments and have tests conducted, you might as well get the best possible overall picture of your thyroid operation. More tests means more information, and more information is going to lead to a better conclusion in nearly every case. Good information is the foundation of good decision making, so give yourself as much info as possible by asking for thorough selection of thyroid tests while you are being evaluated.

Contact Us

In order to get more information regarding thyroid health and how it can impact your life, please feel free to contact us at your convenience. We will be happy to walk you through many of the concepts presented in this book, and we hope that in the end you will be left with a thyroid that is functioning properly and a system that is allowing you to lead the life you desire. Thank you for your time, and here's to good health!